The Tooth Doctor

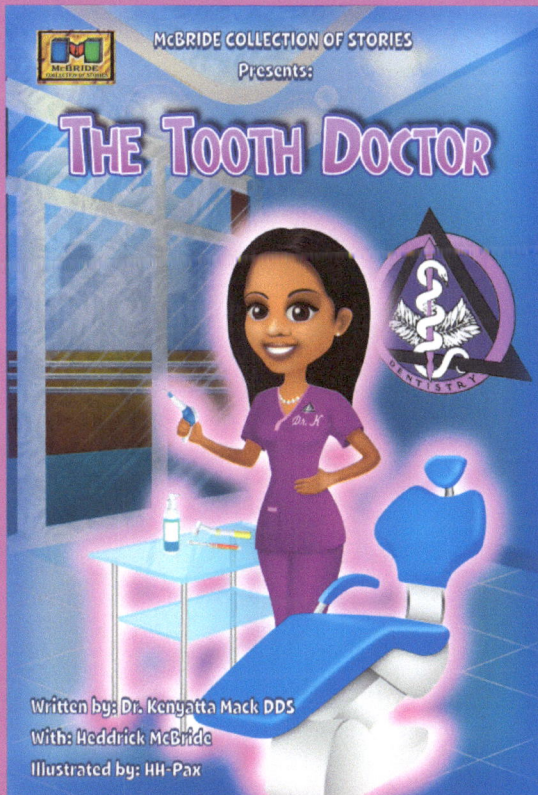

Written by: Dr. Kenyatta Mack DDS

With: Heddrick McBride

Illustrated by: HH-Pax

Edited by: Jill McKellan

The Tooth Doctor

ISBN 10:0615910769
ISBN-13:978-0615910765

About the Author

Dr. Kenyatta Mack DDS (Diva of Dental Smiles)

Dr. Kenyatta Mack grew up in New York City, New York. She attended Marymount College in Tarrytown, New York, where she received her Bachelor of Science in Biology with a minor in Chemistry. Dr. Mack went on to complete her Doctorate of Dental Surgery at Howard University College of Dentistry. Afterward, she completed the Advanced Education in General Dentistry Residency at Metrohealth Hospital Center in Cleveland, Ohio, and a Mini-Pediatric Residency at the University of Maryland in Baltimore, Maryland.

Dr. Mack has been practicing dentistry for over 16 years and is an esteemed member of the following organizations: The American Dental Association, New York State Dental Association, National Dental Association, American Association of Women Dentists, and The American Academy of Pediatric Dentistry. In 2011, Dr. Mack was bestowed the honor of being one of America's Top Dentists.

Dr. Mack is the proud parent of two daughters, Heather Simone and Halle Alexis. In her spare time, she enjoys traveling, reading, and spending time with her family.

Dedication

First and foremost I want to thank God for all the blessings I have received. This book is dedicated to my beautiful daughters, Heather and Halle. You two mean more to me than the air I breathe;and also to my mother, Sandra Mack;my sister, Kyetha Sweeting;my niece and nephews, Kristin, Kyle, and David;Sterling Mack(no I didn't forget you, smile);my sister-in-law, Veronica Gates;and my girls, Yolette, Neshia, and Charliene.

A special dedication goes to the person that has been my rock and protector (you know who you are). You are such a blessing to me. I can't begin to explain how grateful and thankful I am for you, but this comes close:

"For all those times you stood by me;

For all the truth that you made me see

For all the joy you brought to my life

For all the wrong that you made right

For every dream you made come true

For all the love I found in you

I'll be forever thankful baby

You're the one who held me up

Never let me fall

You're the one who saw me through it all

You were my strength when I was weak

You were my voice when I couldn't speak

You were my eyes when I couldn't see

You saw the best there was in me

Lifted me up when I couldn't reach

You gave me faith 'cause you believed

I'm everything I am

Because you loved me."

Lyrics to *Because You Loved Me* written by Diane Warren and made famous by Celine Dion

I would like to thank my family and friends for their support; especially Earl Christian III — thank you so much for this opportunity. I want to give a special shout out to Darrius Gourdine and Shaunia Carlyle for continuously encouraging me to write a book. The one that you guys want me to write is next (wink).

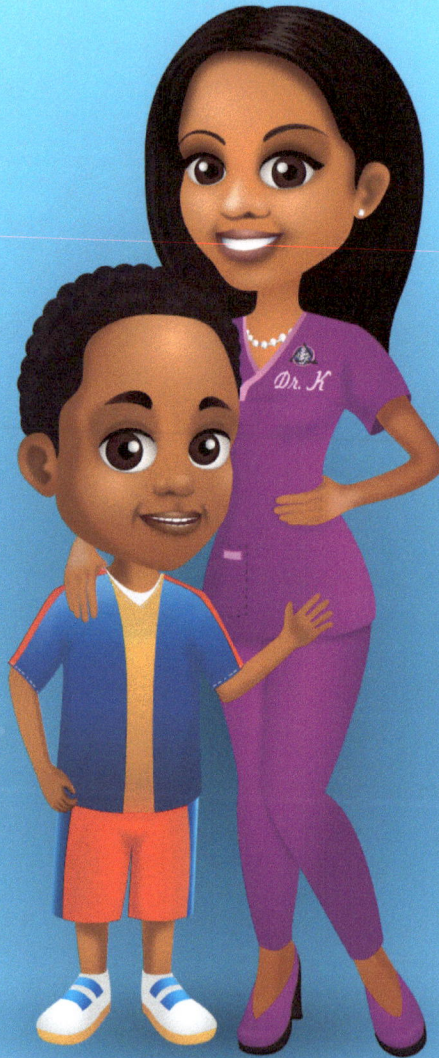

A Day in the Dungeon

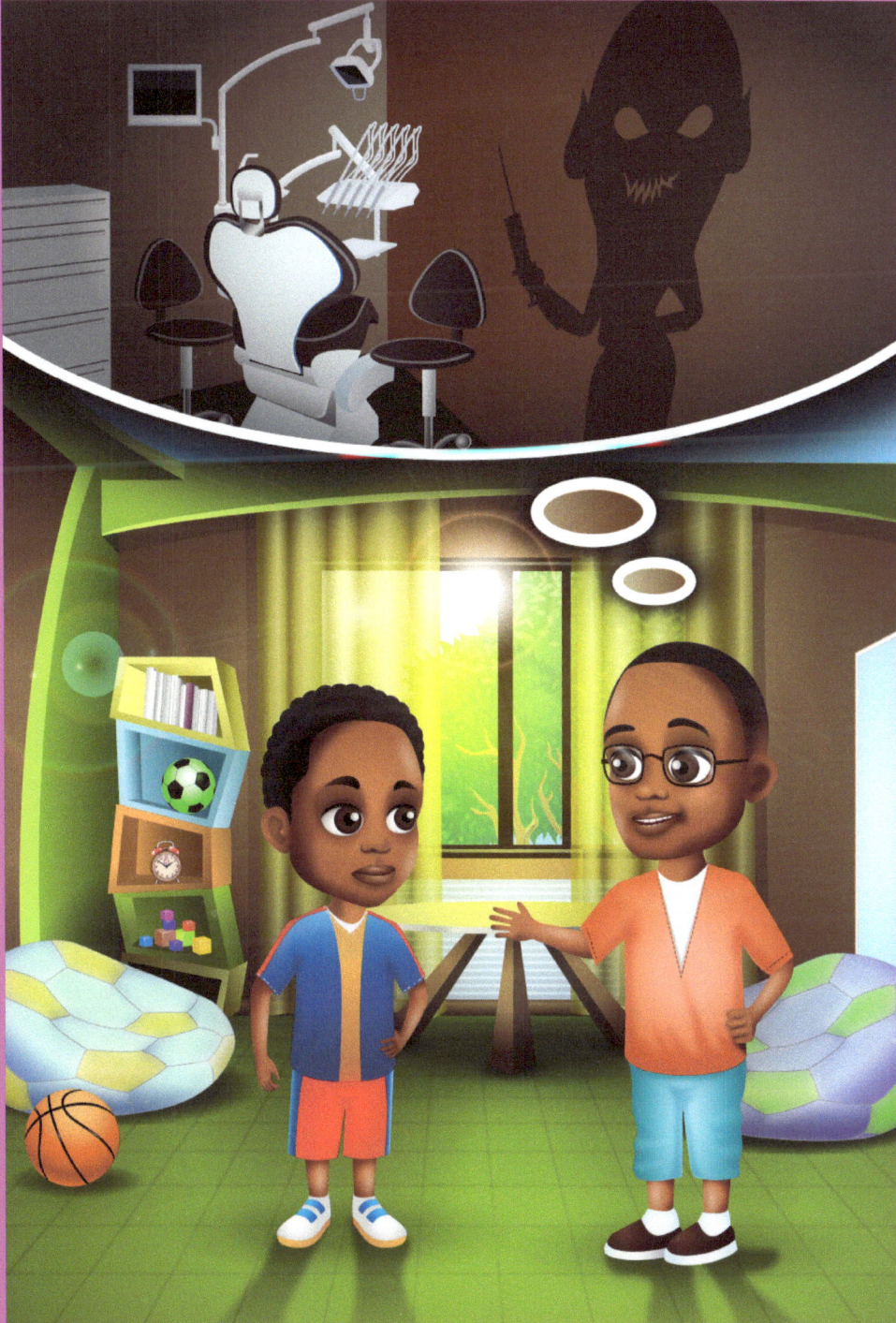

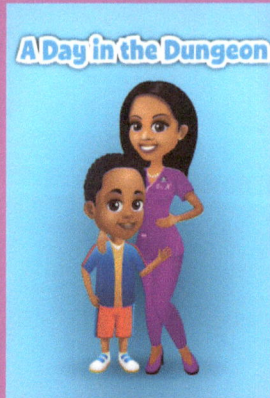

I thought that my dentist office was a dungeon; that's what I was told.

My big brother Kyle said the walls are dark and the rooms are very cold.

He said that the kids are on the first floor, and the cave is underneath.

This is where the evil dentist gives you needles and pulls your teeth.

He said that every kid has to go at least once, but they might not see the cave.

That is only for the ones who act up or misbehave.

I was so terrified that I begged my parents not to take me … not at this time.

My mom laughed and said, "David, everything will be just fine."

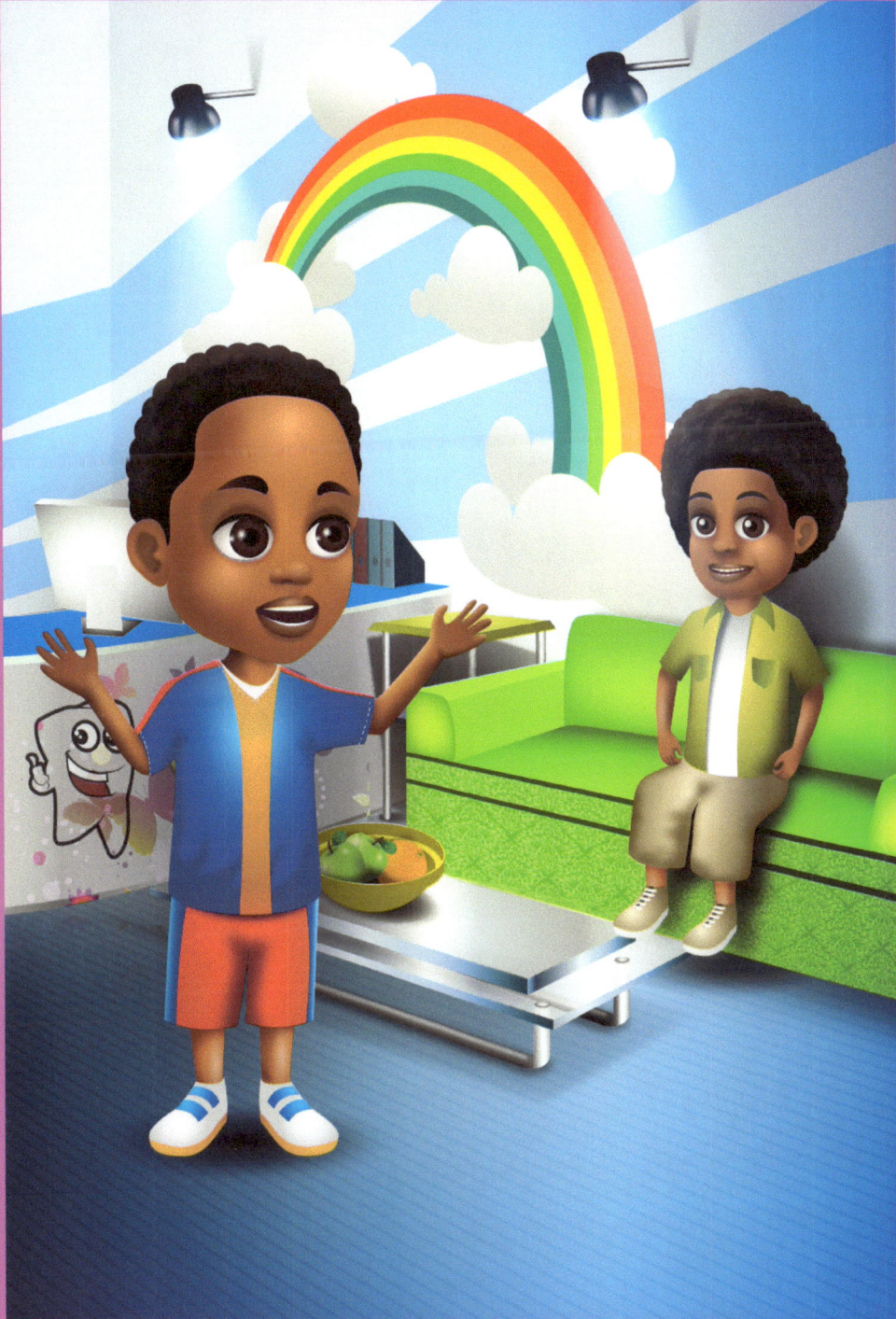

I went in with my hands covering my eyes.

When I took a peak it was a pleasant surprise.

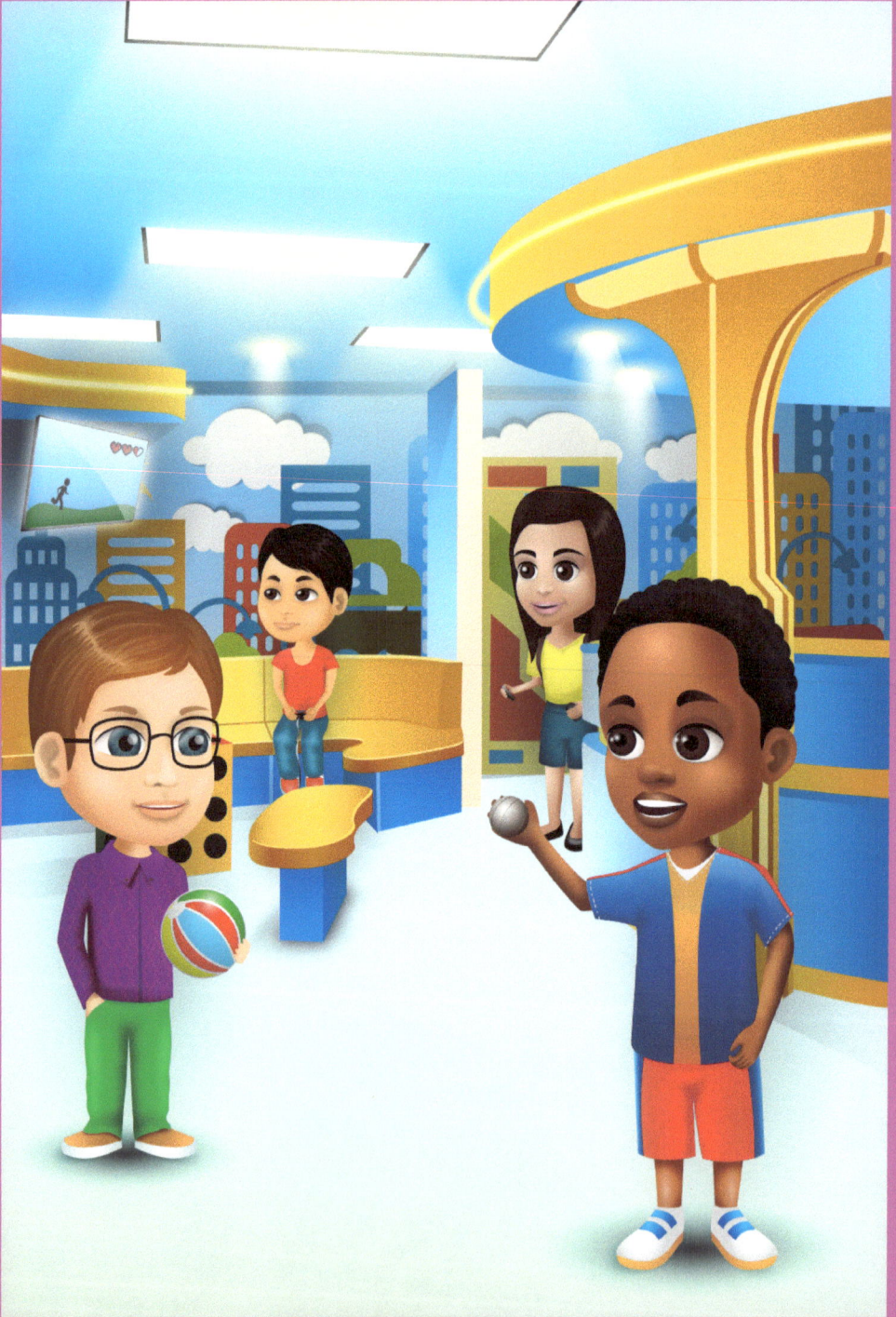

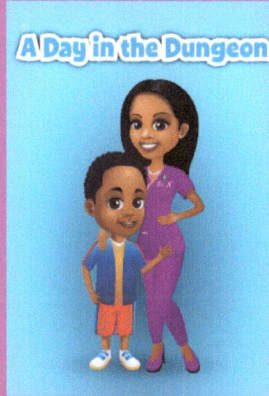

The place that I was so worried about looked like a big place to play.

I saw toys and gadgets; it brightened my day.

There was colorful kids' furniture and bright pictures on the walls.

Kids were laughing and playing video games and throwing a beach ball.

There was a flat screen television and some kids were watching cartoons.

I even saw a few of them blowing up balloons.

One thing I noticed is that everyone had a smile upon their face.

I finally thought that I could be comfortable in this kind of cool place.

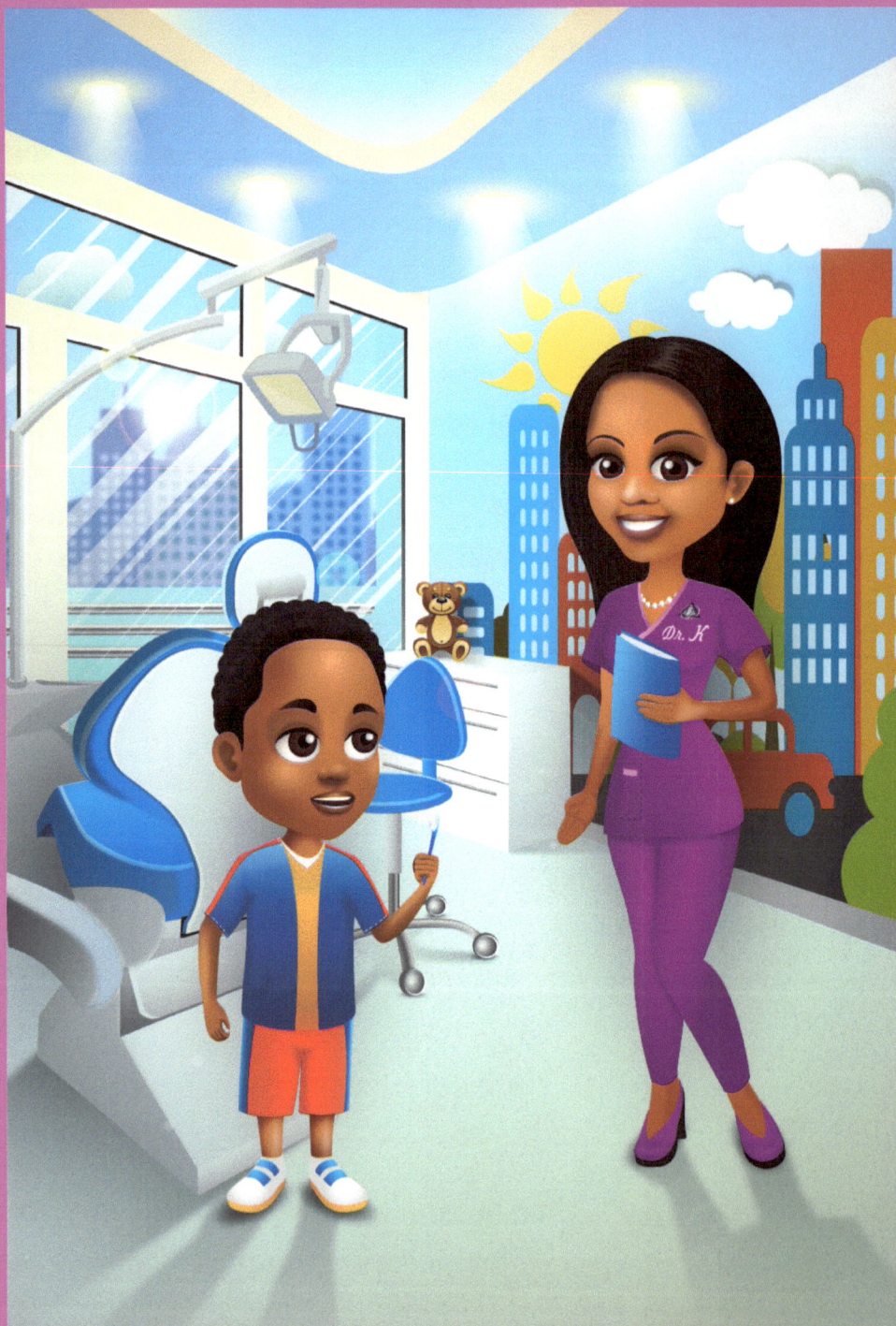

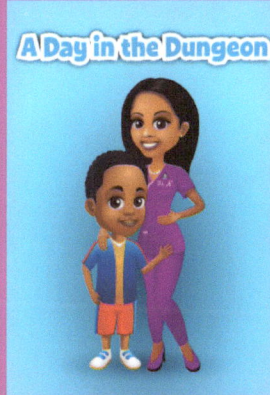

The dentist was named Dr. K and she was nothing like I thought.

She was very friendly, pretty, and she seemed very smart.

Dr. K asked me my name, and also about the things that I like.

She told me a funny story about when she fell off of her bike.

I also met Mr. Thirsty and her special toothbrush.

She even took an x-ray of my teeth. That didn't bother me much.

At the end of my visit, Dr. K asked me if I had any questions.

She gave me some stickers and a new toothbrush for completing my first session.

My day in the dungeon had a very happy end.

My teeth are healthy and Dr. K is my new friend.

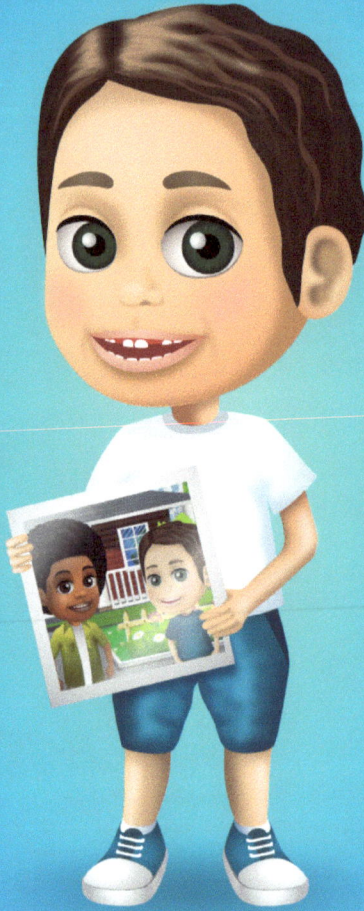

Goodbye Baby Teeth

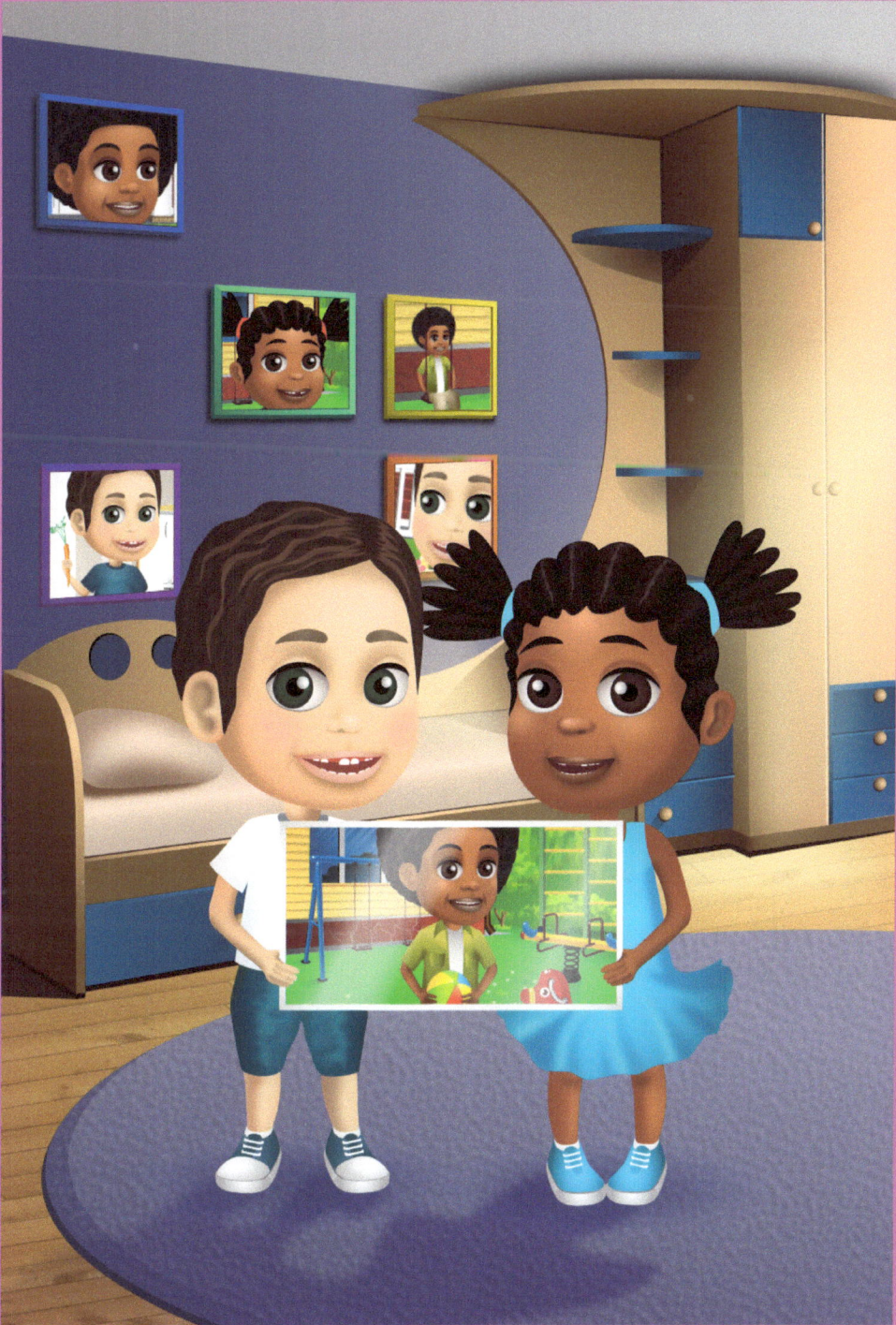

The Tooth Doctor

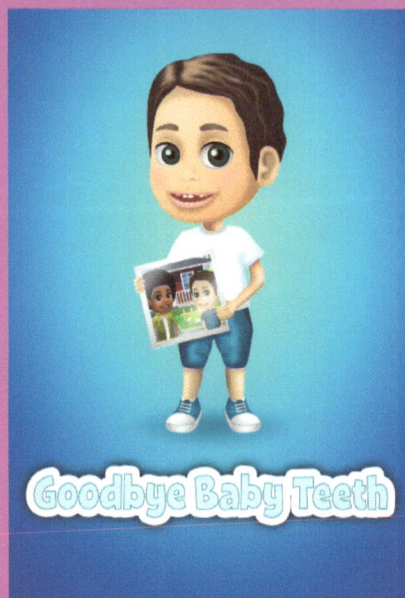

Baby teeth are the first ones that we will grow.

They are responsible for the bright smiles that toddler's show.

Baby teeth are important for proper chewing and eating.

They shape our jaw and help us with our speaking.

We all lose our baby teeth during our childhood ages.

They seem to fall out in four different stages.

Usually by age six or seven we will lose our first tooth.

The first sign of this is when it becomes wobbly and loose.

Between seven and eight, we will lose a few more.

They won't hurt that much, but our gums may be sore.

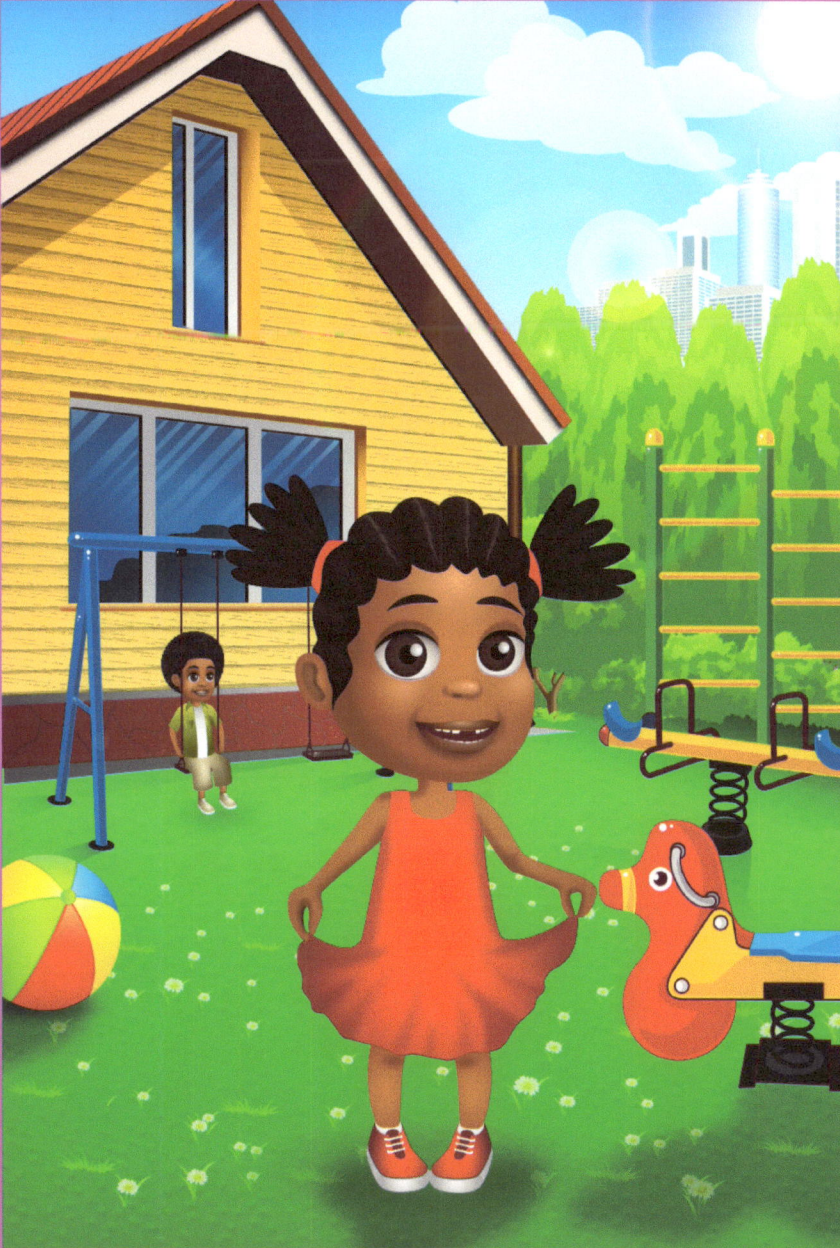

Foods that require chewing and biting may be harder to eat.

You may need to chop it up or cut it into a small piece.

When we turn nine and until we are about twelve, we will lose the rest of the teeth; it's the final stage.

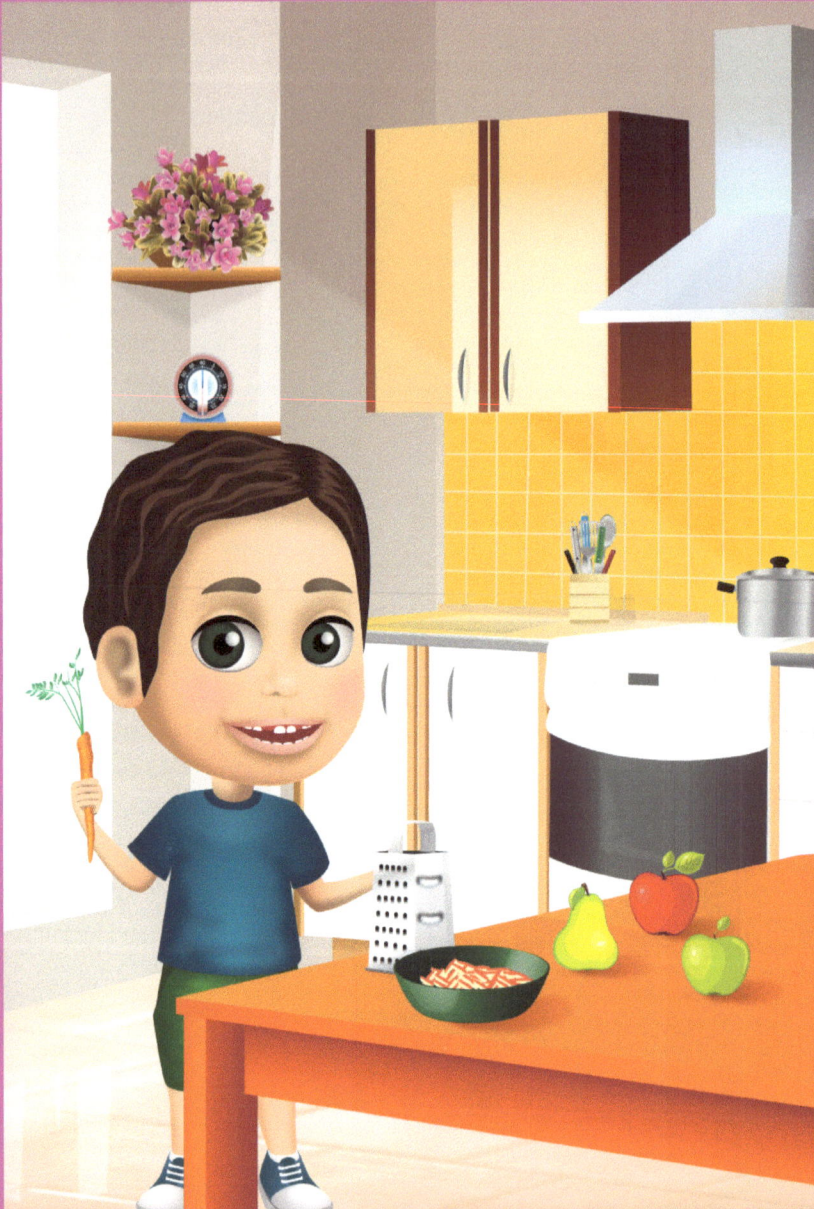

To ensure our new teeth grow in healthy it takes good dental habits.

We still need to brush, floss, and eat healthy foods like carrots.

Saying goodbye to baby teeth is not a bad thing.

Many funny pictures and memories it does bring.

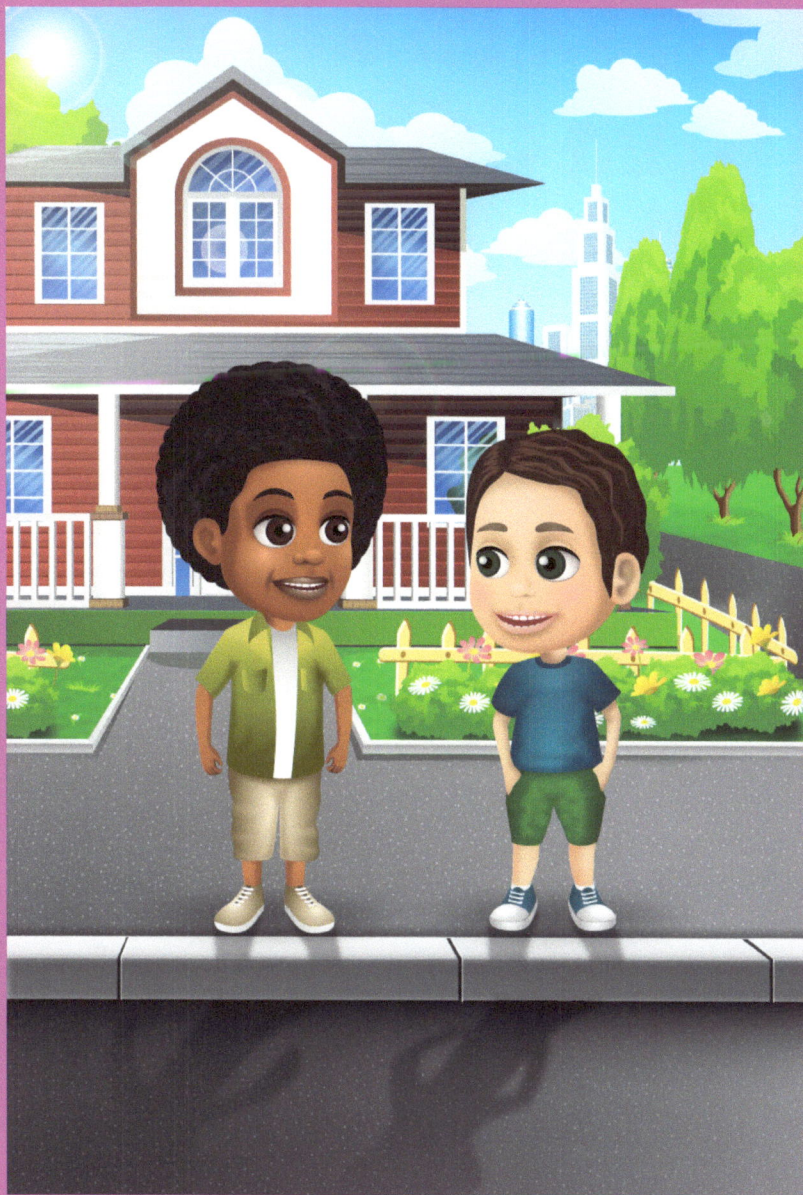

We have to treat our new teeth right so that they become stronger.

They will come in healthy and last much longer.

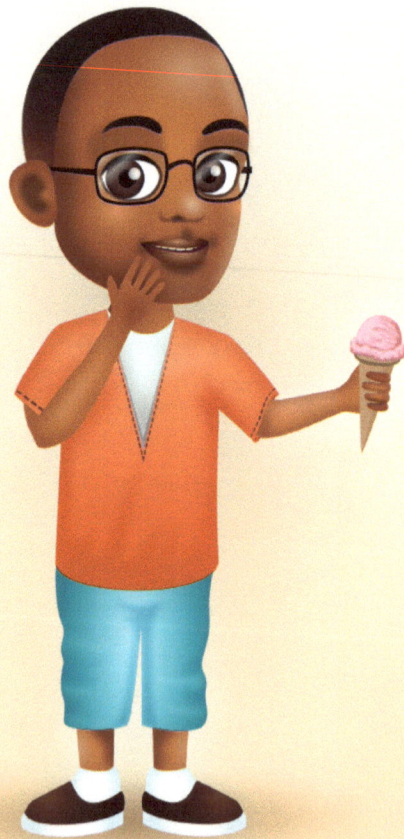

Let's keep away from Cavities

Let's keep away from cavities because they are not pleasant.

Many people get them and they are not a welcome present.

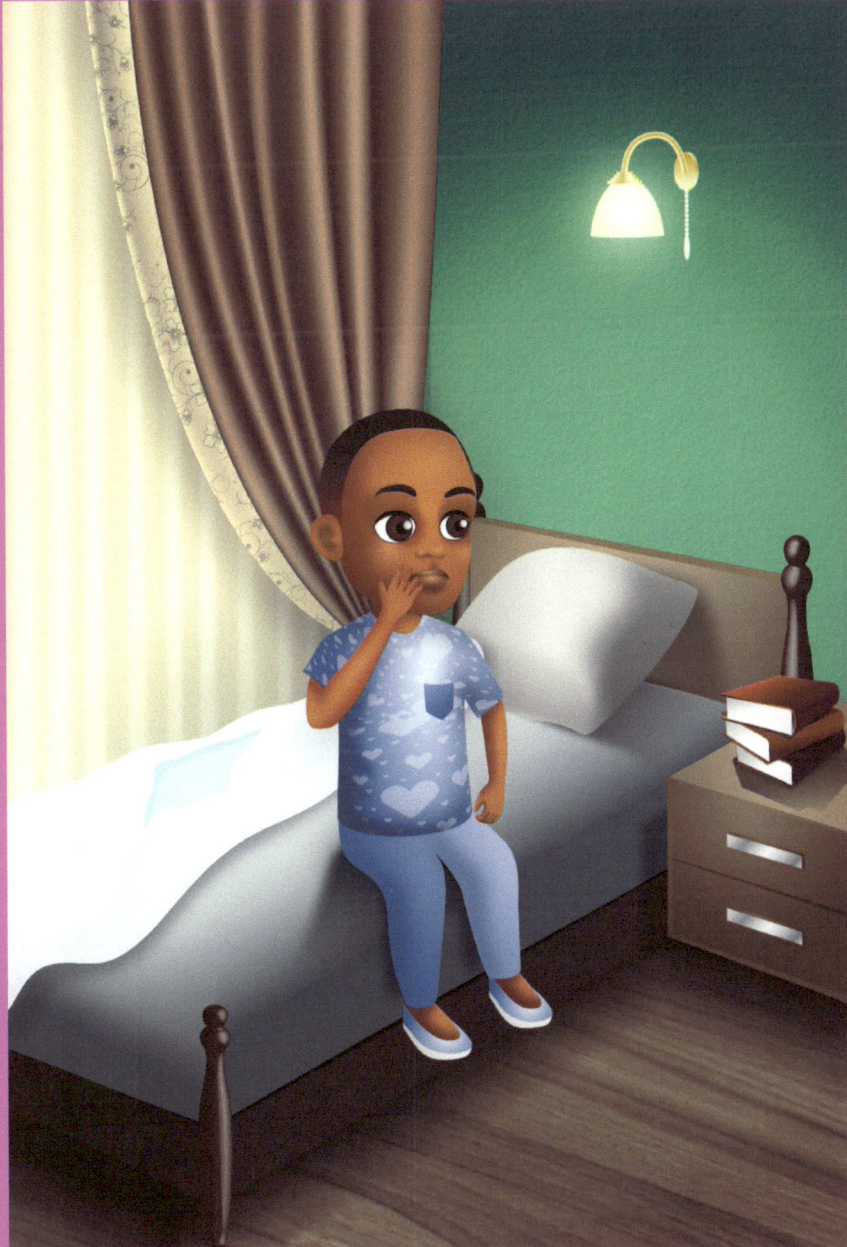

Cavities are decay that is formed by bacteria in our teeth.

They hurt so much that they even make it hard to sleep.

They are formed when we have sugary foods or drinks.

We may not be cleaning our mouths as well as we think.

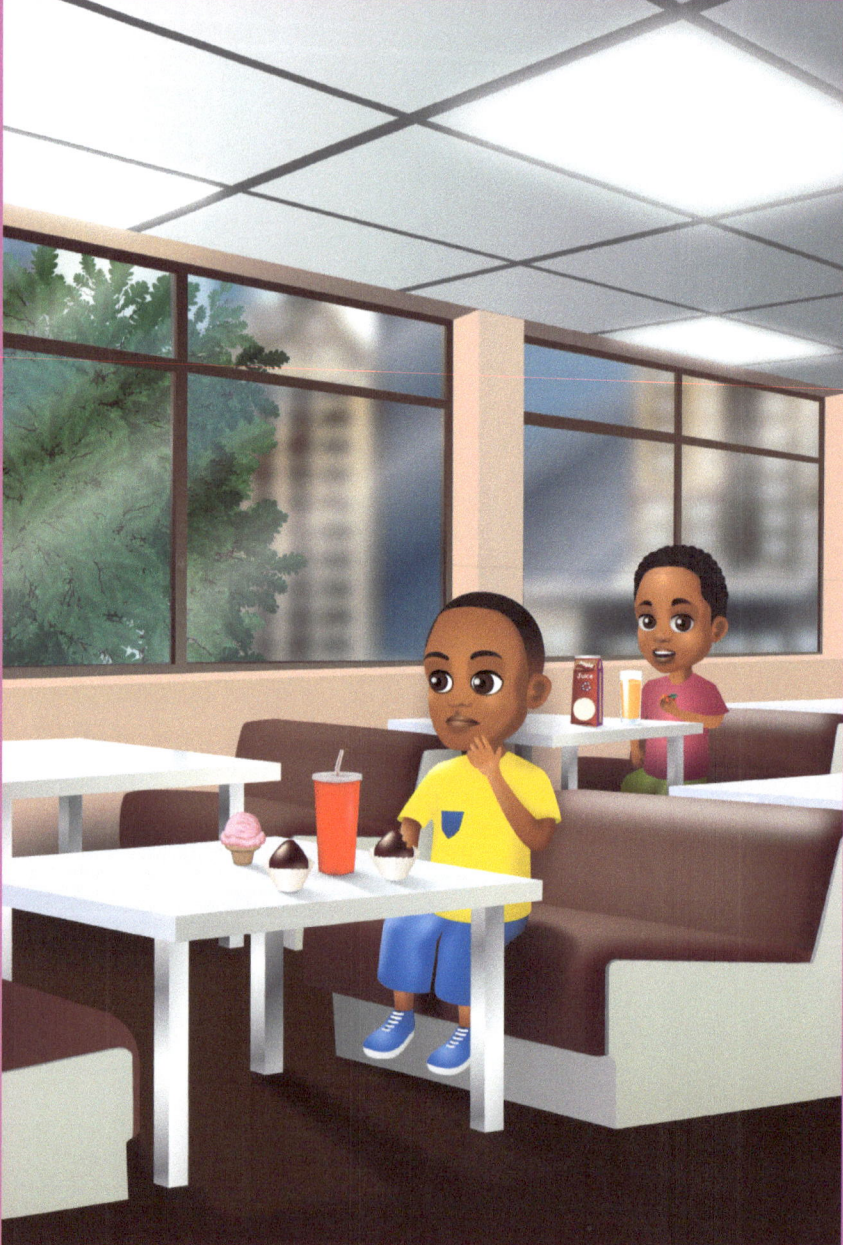

The sugar turns into acid that eats through our teeth.

It forms holes that may burn or hurt when you eat.

Here are some ways to keep cavities away so that we won't have to have these unpleasant days.

We should brush our teeth properly at least two times a day. This will wash the sugar and food away.

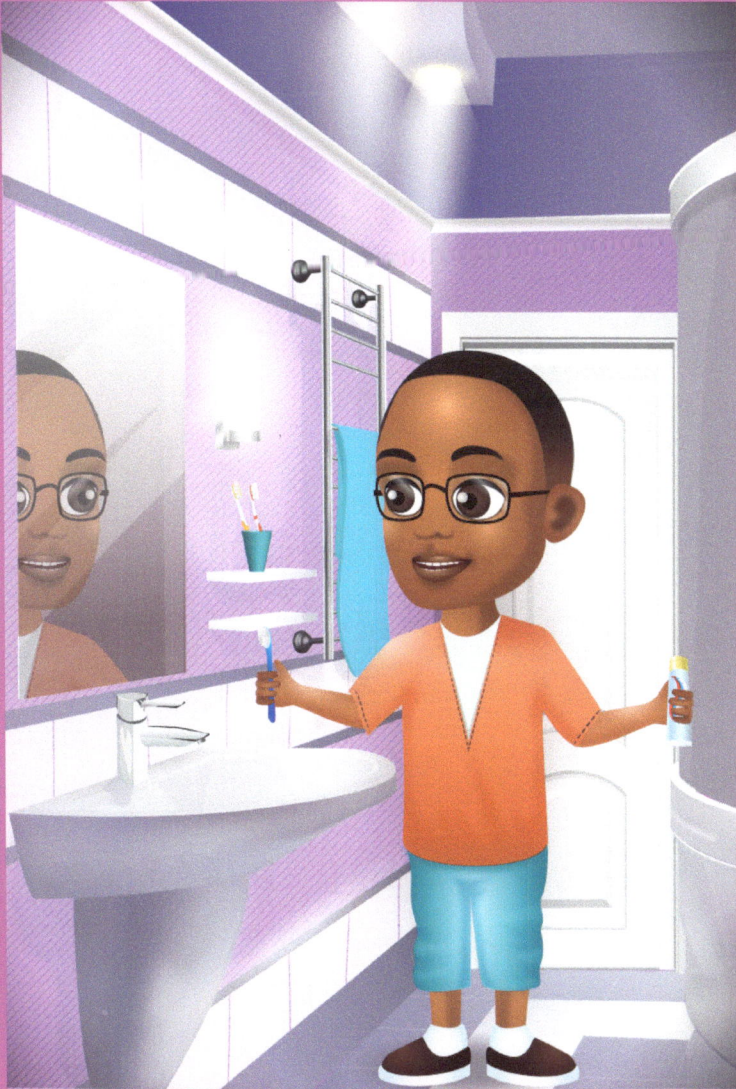

Using floss every night before bed will give us more reach.

It will help to get the small things out from in between our teeth.

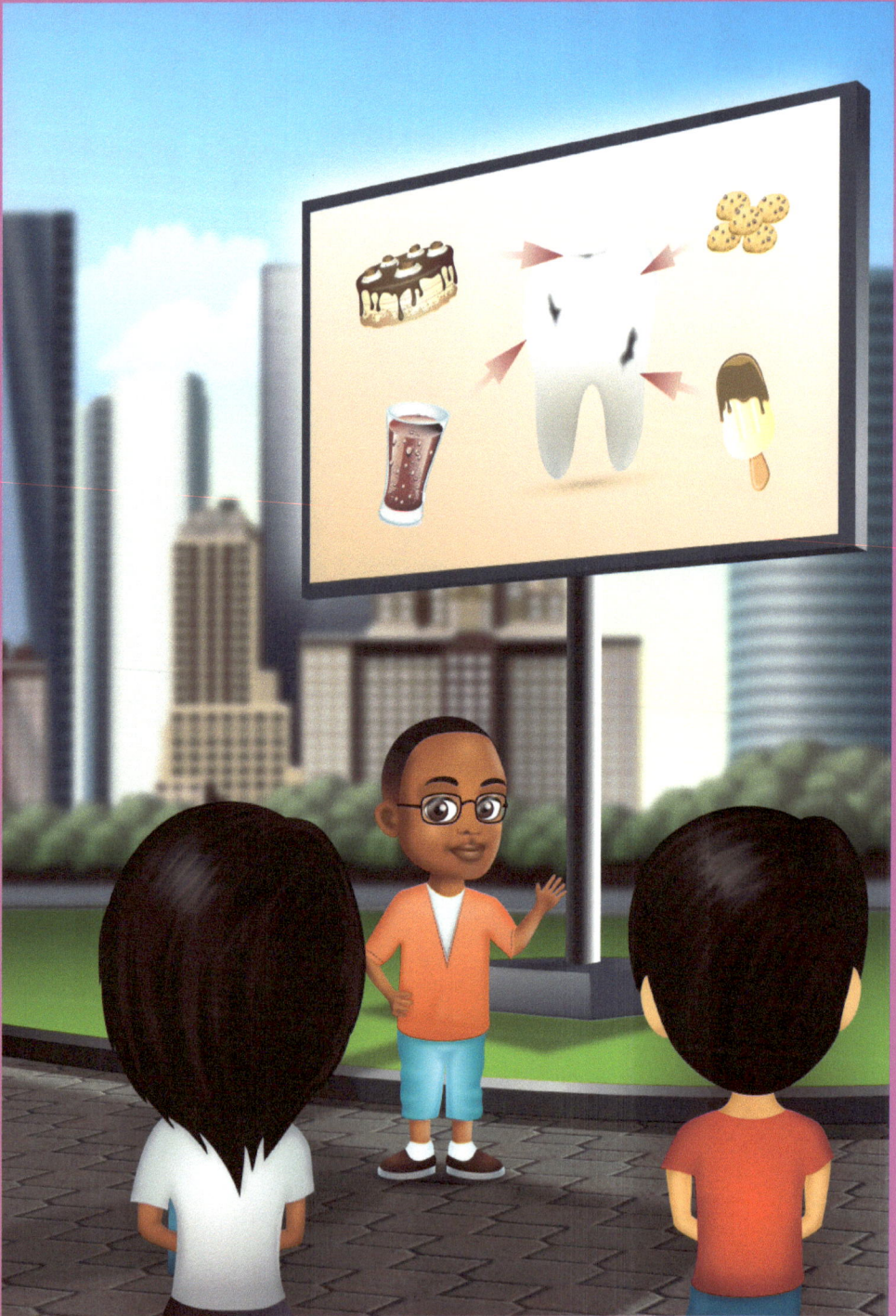

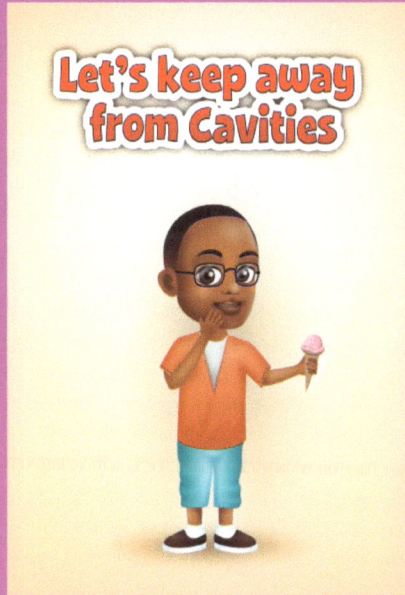

Let's cut back on the amount of candy that we eat and sugary liquids we drink.

These simple things help more than we think.

Water is good for us, but we still need fluoride too.

This is something that the dentist can provide you.

We should also schedule regular appointments with our dentist and pay attention.

They will check for cavities and teach us about cavity prevention.

If we follow these steps each and every day, we will keep the cavities away.

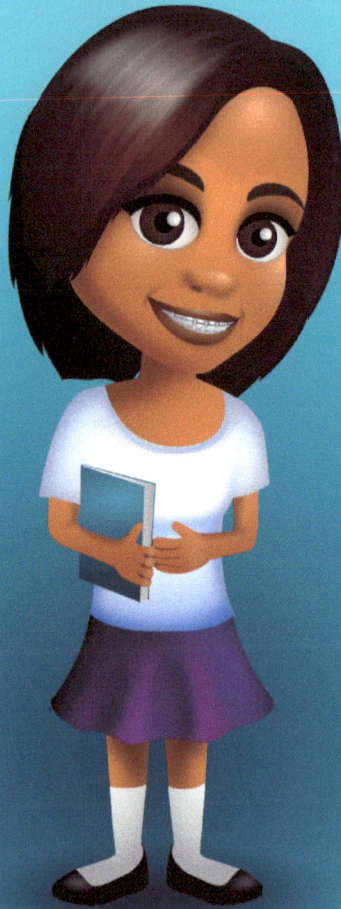

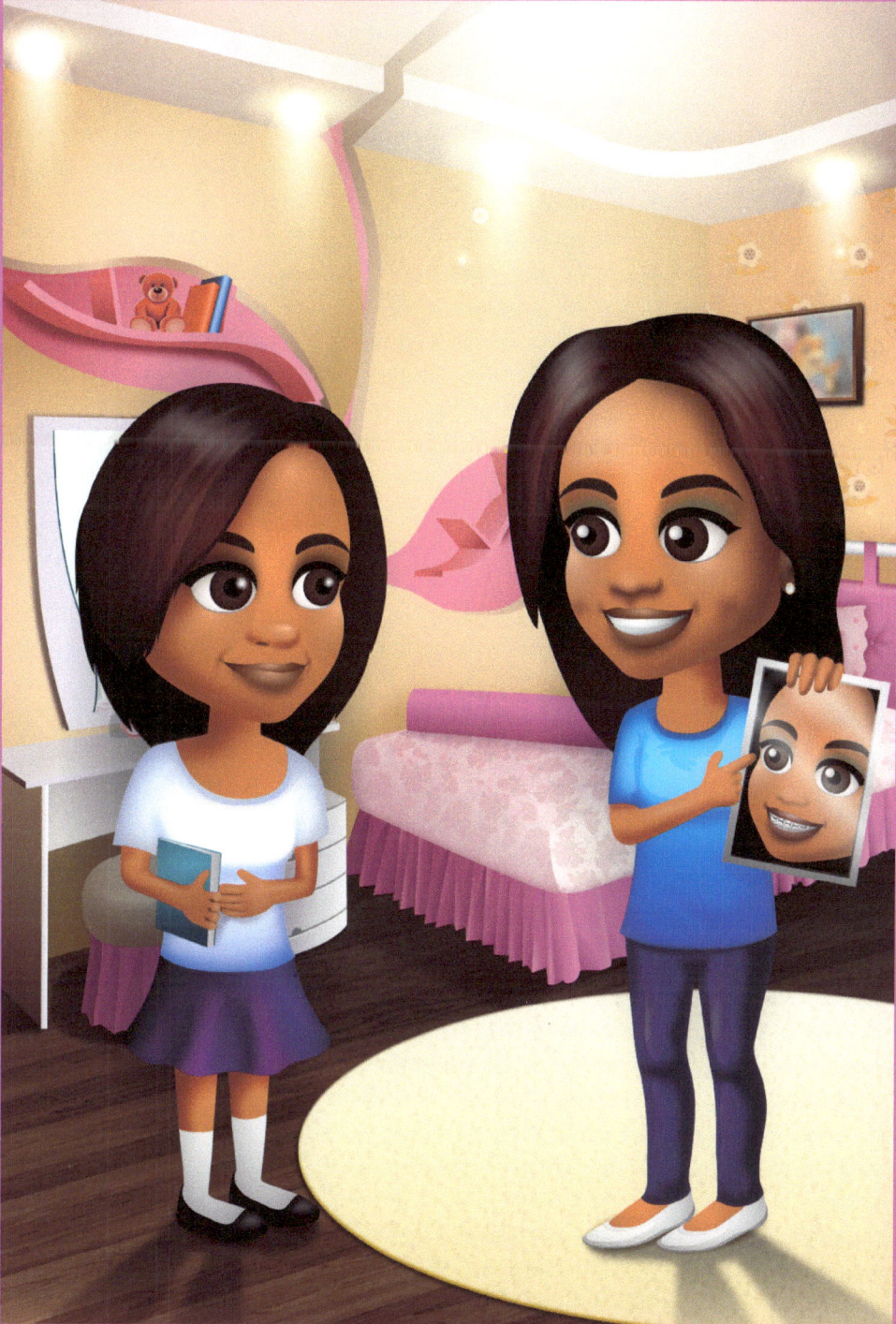

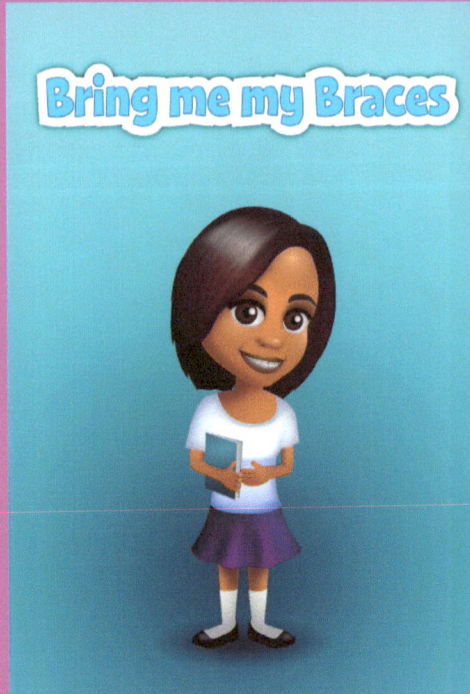

Bring me my braces because I have seen what they can do.

My sister Heather once had a crooked smile, but now it looks brand new.

I asked her how she did it and she said by wearing braces.

Braces have helped many kids have happy smiling faces.

Braces main job are to make your teeth straight and upright.

You may start with crooked teeth or an overbite.

They go on and around your teeth to make them stay in place.

This helps them line up correctly with your jaw and the rest of your face.

There are different types of braces that I may be able to use.

Metal, plastic, and ceramic are some kinds that I may choose.

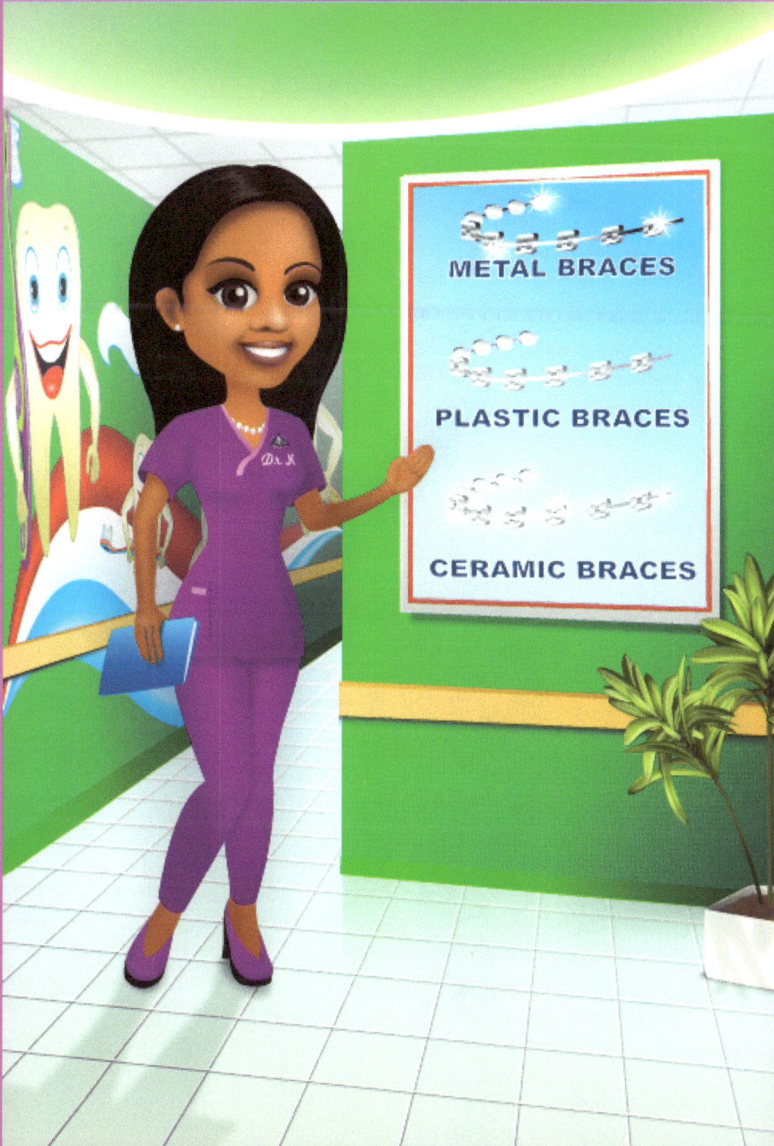

There are braces that are clear, but they are only suitable for some.

People like these because you can hide them from everyone.

I learned that having braces means that I have to treat them with special care.

Avoiding popcorn, gum, and sticky candy is important; it may get stuck in there.

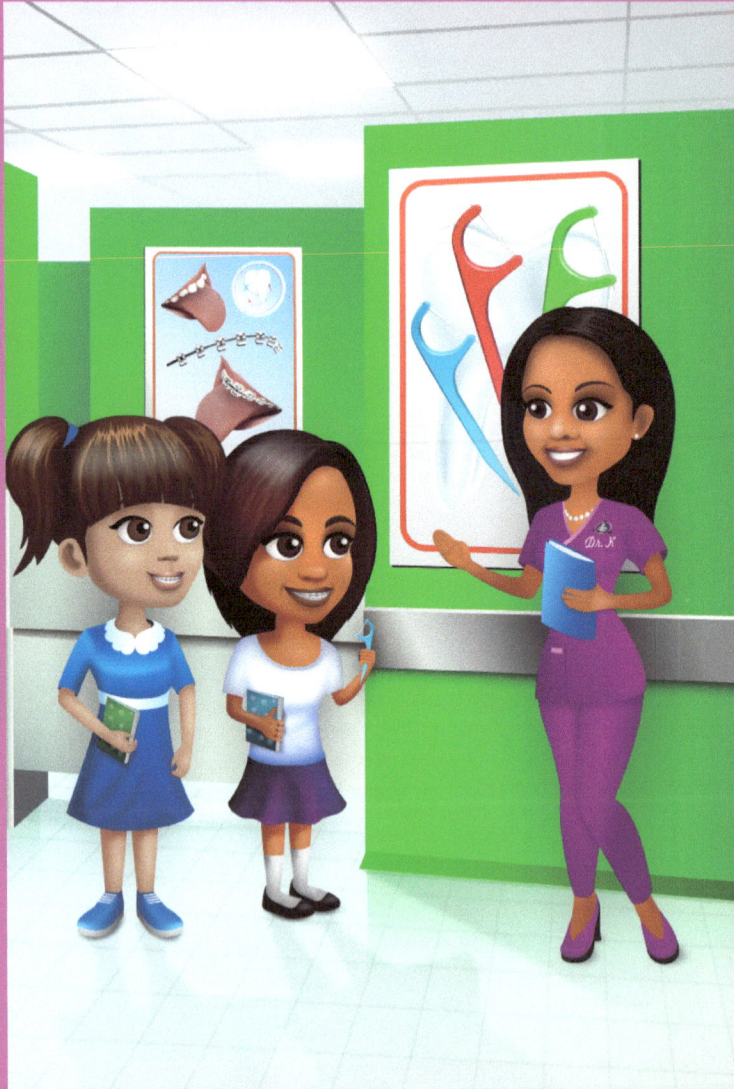

Making sure I brush after meals and floss is still something I should do;

Just to make sure that I don't get any cavities that are new.

Dr. K told me not to be embarrassed or ashamed to wear them.

If people make jokes, then just pretend not to hear them.

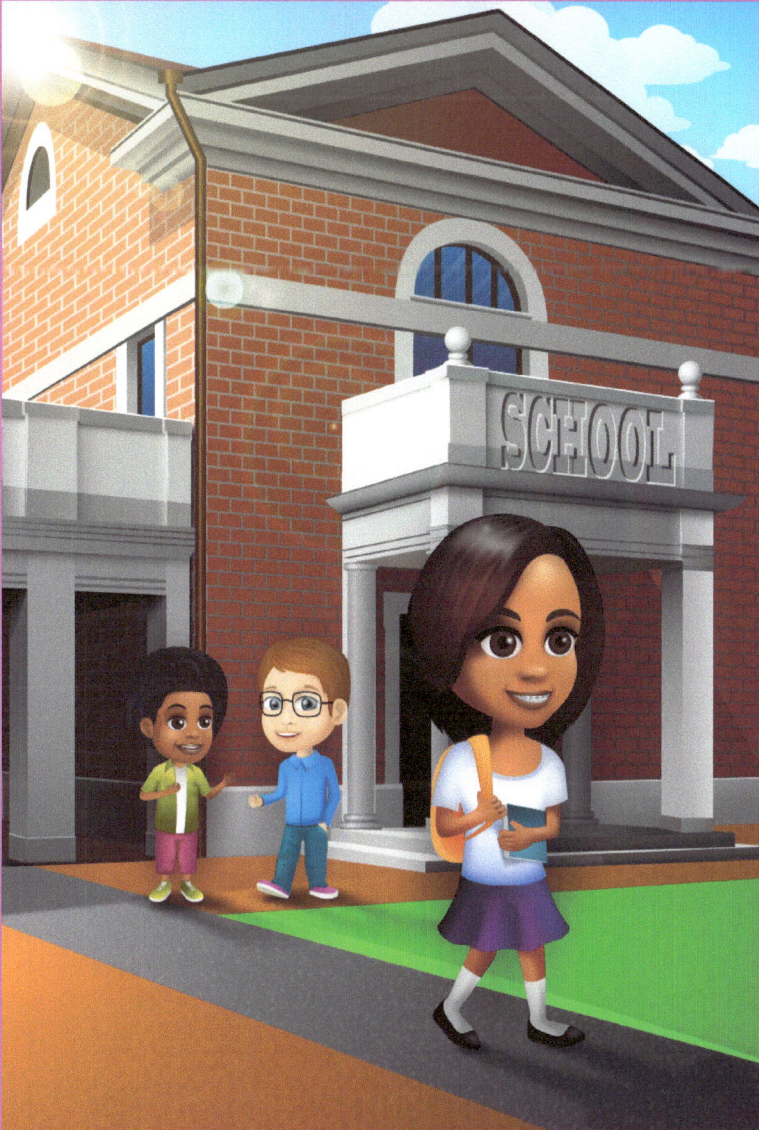

She said, "Halle, in two years you will end up with teeth that are perfect and straight.

Bring me my braces now because I can't wait.

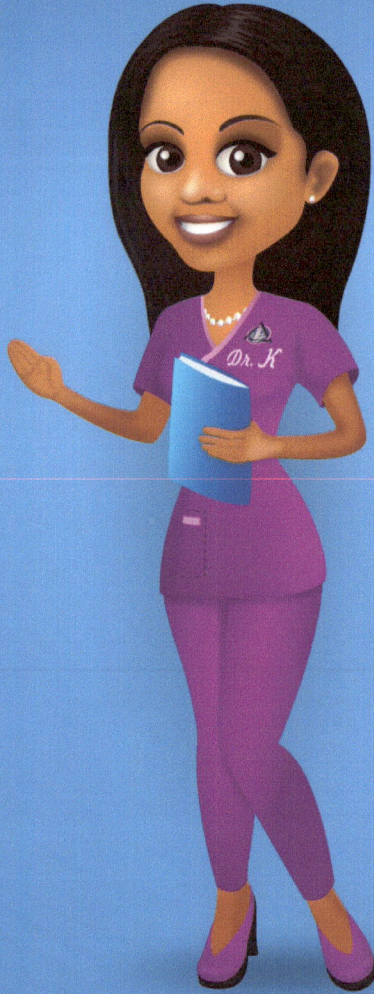

Foods for our Teeth

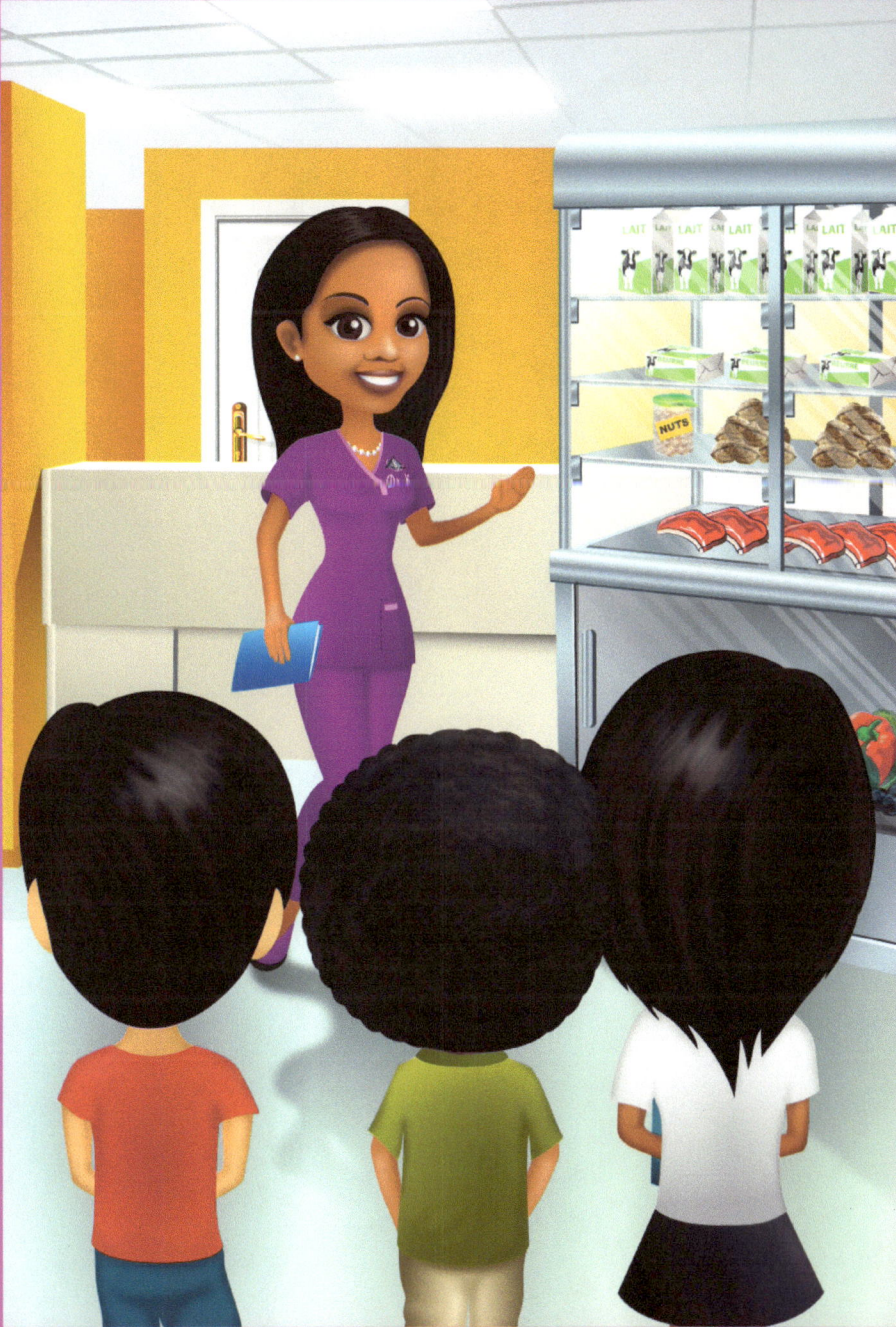

Eating the right types of foods can keep our gums and teeth in good condition.

It's a great way to keep the cavities missing.

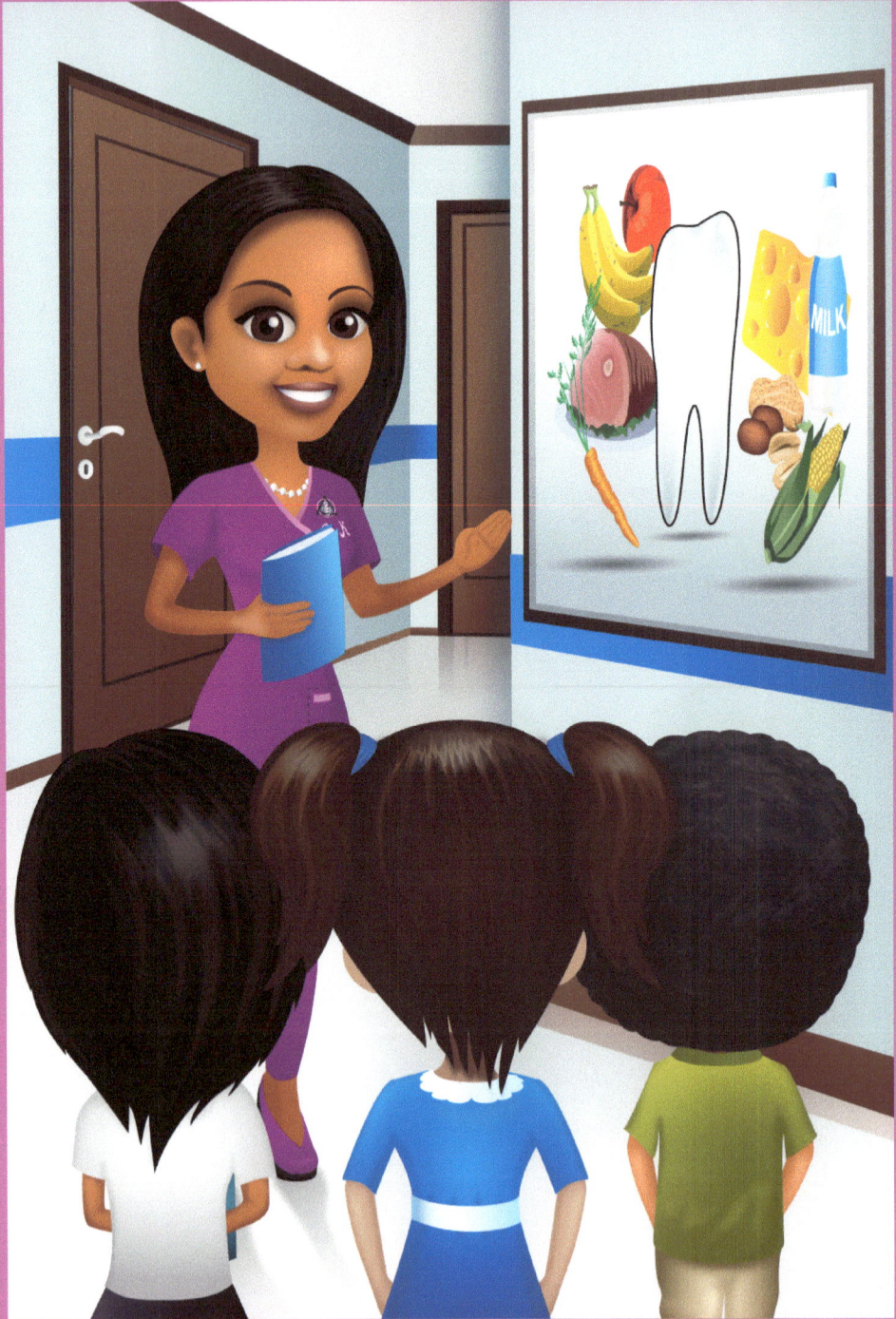

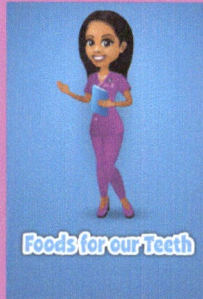

We need to learn which foods we should limit and which to avoid.

If we don't take this seriously then our teeth may be destroyed.

Cheese, milk, red meat, and nuts provide Vitamin D.

This helps spread calcium throughout our body.

Calcium helps to strengthen our gums, teeth, and jaw bone.

It also helps keep gum disease out of your mouth, your food's home.

Foods like apples, pears, and vegetables protect against tooth decay.

They provide saliva which protects by washing extra food and acid away.

There are some healthy foods that may not always be good for our mouth.

Fruits like oranges, tomatoes, and lemons have acid, so only eat small amounts.

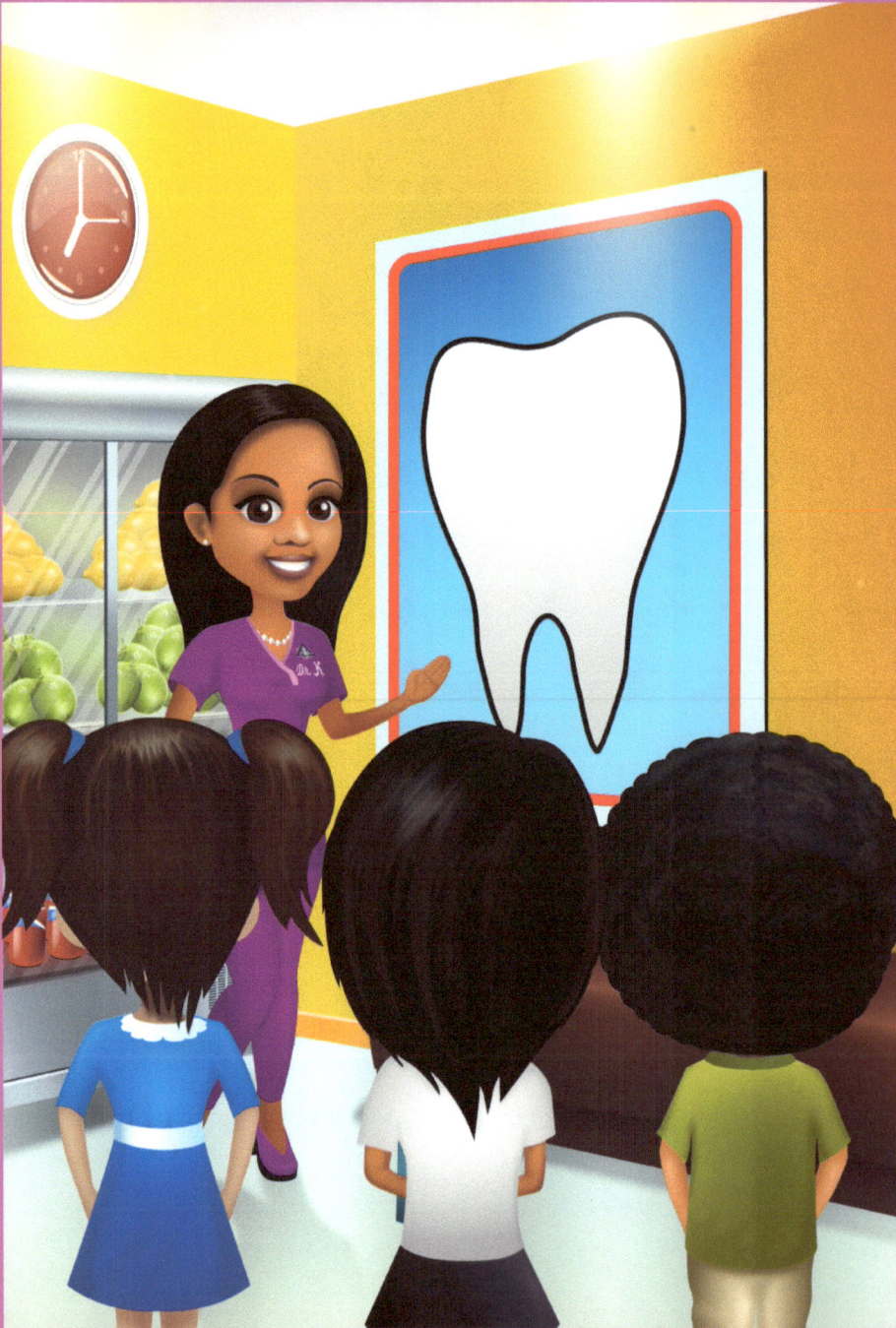

Remember, acid helps destroy our tooth enamel and weakens our gums.

Then before you know it, new cavities may come.

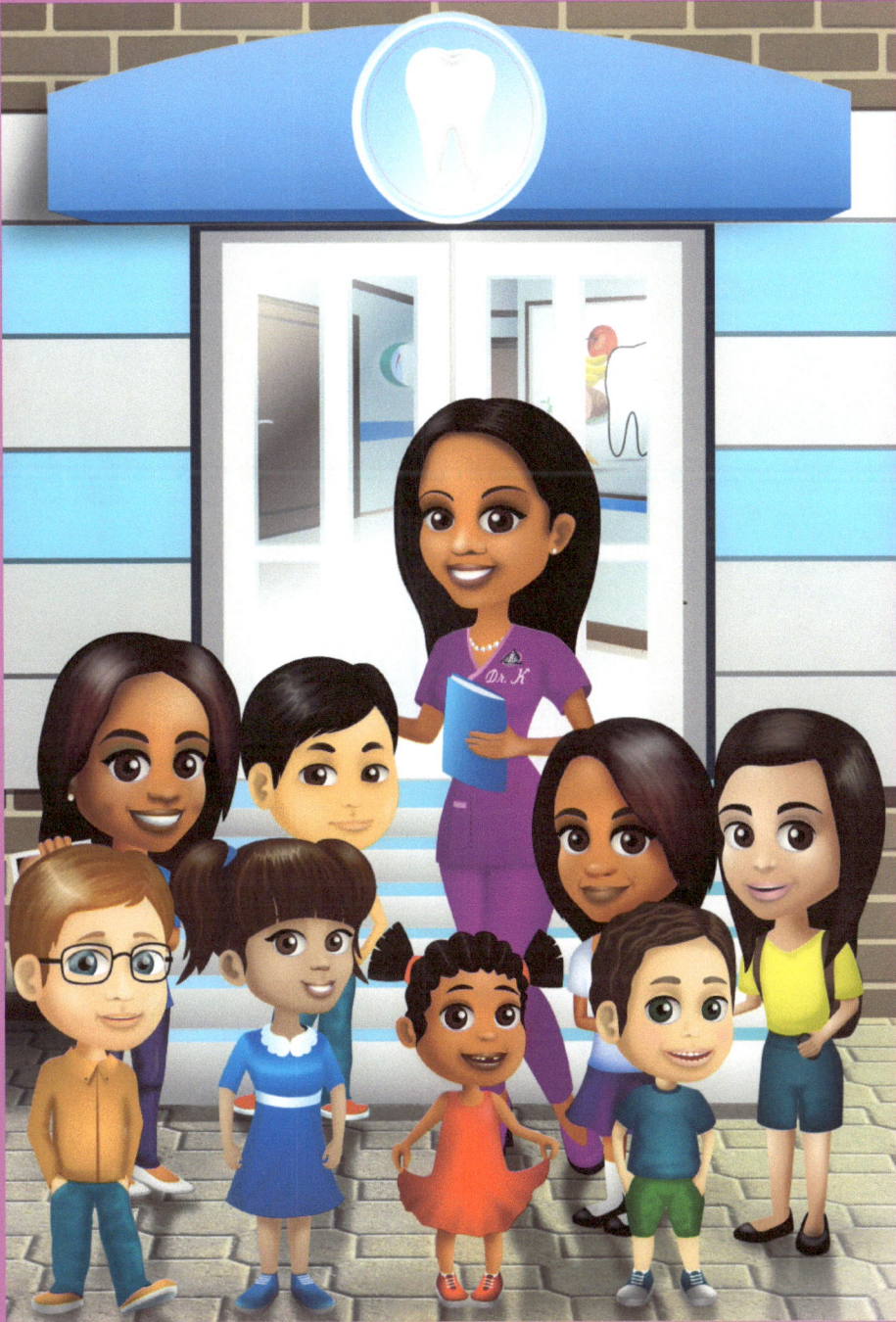

This is a quick lesson on taking care of your teeth.

They are affected by all the things that we drink and the foods that we eat.

Visit www.mcbridestories.com for more titles.

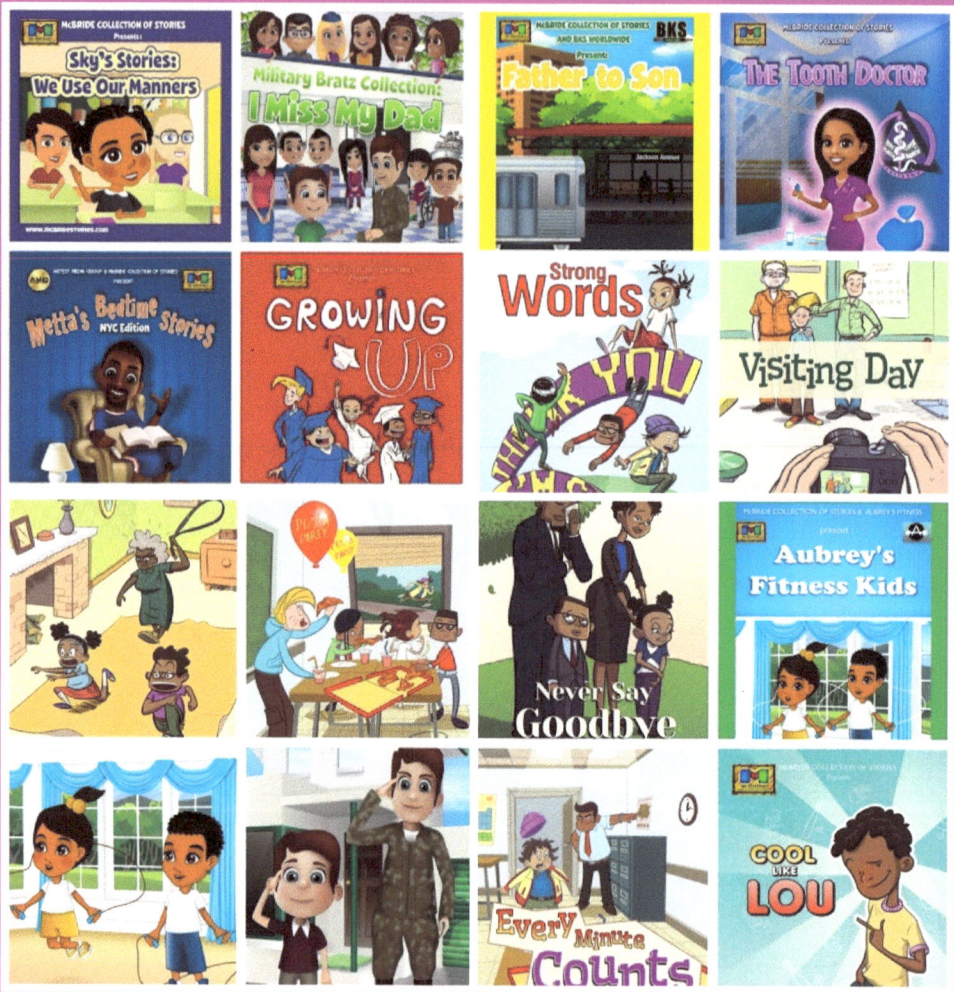

www.ingramcontent.com/pod-product-compliance
Lightning Source LLC
Chambersburg PA
CBHW060834270326
41933CB00002B/79